This Mediterr___ ___t
Tracker

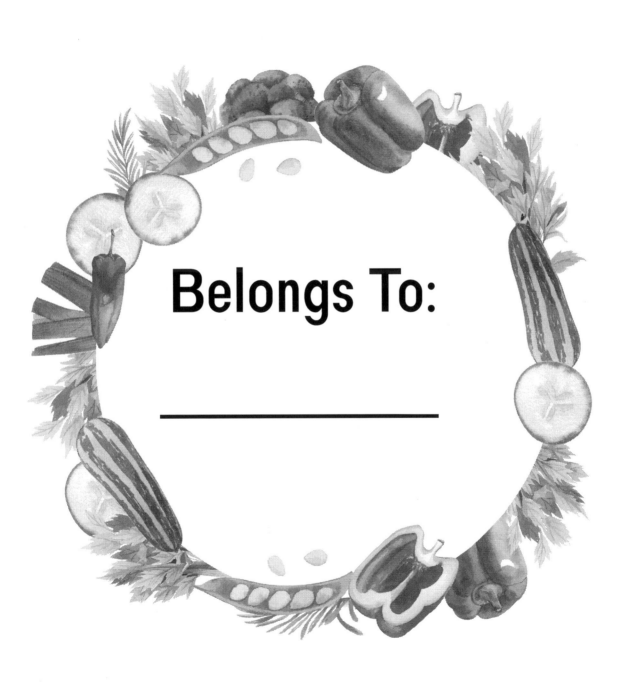

Belongs To:

_____

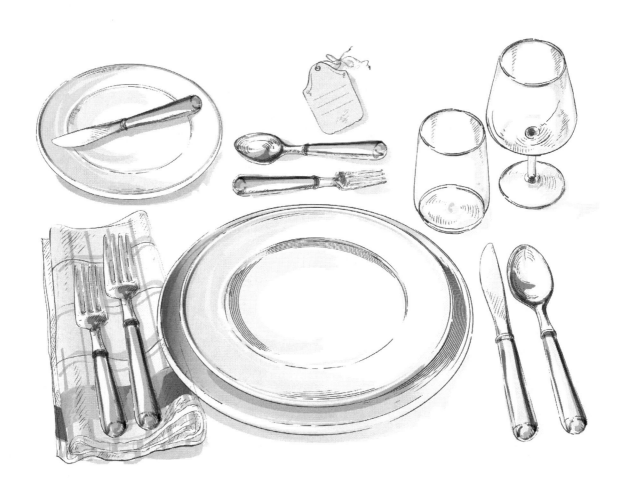

Mediterranean Diet Overview

Dieting that word, we all love to hate, but unfortunately for many of us there is a vital need to keep trying to find the right combination that we can utilize to achieve our goals but also enjoy the food without feeling deprived.

I should know having tried so many different food regimes that promised the earth and either made me feel ill or deprived. I thought I had found the solution with Keto and whilst that helped in the short term, it wasn't sustainable for me in the long term.

What I wanted was an eating lifestyle that would enable me to feel better, give my body the nutrients it needed but still allow for occasional treats and foods I enjoyed without sabotaging what I had done to date.

This is why I am so passionate about the Mediterranean lifestyle and it is a lifestyle, not a diet, once you get on board with this way of healthy eating you won't want to go back.

If someone had told me a month ago, I wouldn't have my lifelong cravings for sweets, that I would have more energy and overall feel so much better I would have been very skeptical.

But here I am saying those are the things that happened for me, and let's not forget the weight loss, what's that adage? Slow and steady wins the race.

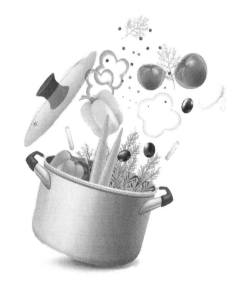

So, you might be asking at this point what exactly is this way of eating, quite simply it is based round the eating habits and customs of the countries that surround the Mediterranean Sea. This is a lifestyle that revels in healthy food and vegetables, olive oil, red wine and so much more.

The concept is derived from the eating habits and meal customs of the countries that are based around the Mediterranean Sea where the people enjoy olive oil, red wine, delicious vegetables and more.

What Is This Book For?

I won't elaborate any further on in depth details of the Mediterranean diet as that is not the intent of this book and searching online or your local bookstore will result in a plethora of information from far more informed and detailed sources than my personal experiences.

So, What Is This Book For?

This book is intended to be used as a tool to help you manage the start of your own Mediterranean Lifestyle journey. It is based on the method I used to get myself into a routine and become familiar with my new lifestyle.

When you first start any diet, it takes time to adjust and learn what you can and can't eat, and things like portion sizes and best combinations. Then you need to be aware of calories counts, carbs, fats and proteins etc. Now those things of course are all manageable these days with apps and online calculators, but some of us just like to have something manual we can record and monitor our progress in.

This book gives you a way to organize and structure your first 4 weeks until you get used to this style of eating and it becomes second nature.

There are a range of pages to help keep track of allowed foods, blank favorite foods pages for you to add your own preferences, blank shopping lists, 4 blank weekly plans with daily tracking days, and other pages to enable monitoring exercise and weight loss.

I have also added blank pages for your favorite recipes at the back of the book as I found it convenient to keep everything together in one place rather than various places on the internet or numerous notes.

This is **NOT** a cookbook full of recipes nor is it full of detailed plans and explanations about the Mediterranean lifestyle, but hopefully it will provide you with a useful tool to manage your new adventure to the Mediterranean.

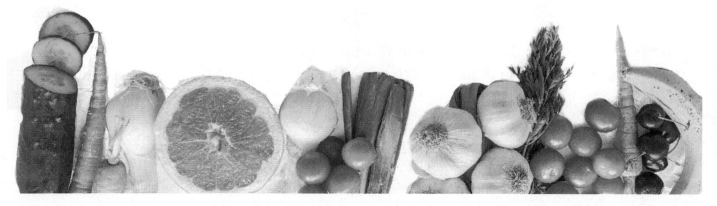

28 Day Challenge

- [ ]
- [ ]
- [ ]
- [ ]
- [ ]
- [ ]
- [ ]
- [ ]
- [ ]
- [ ]
- [ ]
- [ ]
- [ ]
- [ ]
- [ ]
- [ ]
- [ ]
- [ ]

INSPIRATIONAL REMINDERS

STARTED >

FINISHED >

1	2	3	4	5	6	7	8	9	10
11	12	13	14	15	16	17	18	19	20
21	22	23	24	25	26	27	28	29	30

30-DAY MEDITERRANEAN RESULTS

PERSONAL ACCOMPLISHMENTS

Before & After

WEIGHT	WEIGHT
BMI	BMI
BODY FAT	BODY FAT
MUSCLE	MUSCLE
CHEST	CHEST
WAIST	WAIST
HIPS	HIPS
THIGHS	THIGHS
CALF	CALF
BICEP	BICEP
OTHER :	OTHER :
OTHER :	OTHER :

Weight Loss Tracker

MONTHLY GOAL

WEEKLY WEIGHT LOSS TRACKER

DATE:

	BUST				
	WAIST				
	HIPS				
	BICEP				
	THIGH				
	CALF				
	WEIGHT				
TOTAL WEIGHT LOSS >>					

Mediterranean Start Date

Outline your most important fitness goals

Describe how you see yourself in six months

DATE	MEDITERRANEAN WEIGHT LOSS ACTION PLAN		PERSONAL MILESTONES

Mediterranean Allowed Foods

MEATS & FISH

- Anchovies
- Chicken
- Cod
- Lamb
- Shrimp/Prawns
- Mussels
- Salmon
- Sardines/Tuna

VEGGIES

- Avocado
- Asparagus
- Artichoke
- Broccoli
- Cauliflower
- Brussel Sprouts
- Cabbage
- Celery/Onions

VEGGIES

- Cucumber
- Tomatoes
- Peppers/Lettuce
- Green Beans
- Zucchini
- Mushrooms
- Spinach/Kale
- Olives/Eggplant

FRUITS

- Apples/Watermelon
- Oranges/Lemons
- Bananas
- Blueberries
- Dates/Figs
- Grapefruit
- Grapes/Blackberries
- Strawberries

DAIRY

- Eggs
- Feta Cheese
- Goat Cheese
- Parmesan/Ricotta
- Greek Yogurt
- Almond Milk
- Cashew Milk
- Skim Milk (Limited)

CONDIMENTS

- Balsamic Vinegar
- Olive Oil
- Coconut Butter
- Hummus
- Nut Oils
- Pesto/Tahini
- Red Wine Vinegar
- Sun Dried Tomatoes

HERBS & SPICES

- Basil
- Dill
- Rosemary
- Cinnamon
- Oregano
- Parsley
- Capers
- Thyme

HERBS & SPICES

- Garlic
- Salt & Pepper
- Onion Salt
- Paprika
- Cumin
- Chili Pepper
- Basil
- Ginger

BAKING

- Almond Flour
- Almond Meal
- Cashew Flour
- Oat Fiber
- Psyllium Husk
- Wholemeal Flour
- Flax meal

GRAINS

- Barley
- Brown Rice
- Bulgar
- Couscous
- Farro
- Quinoa
- Whole Grain Bread
- Wole Grain Pasta

DRINKS

- Water
- Coffee
- Tea
- Broth
- Coconut Water
- Wine (Limited)

LEGUMES/NUTS

- Cannellini Beans
- Chickpeas
- Kidney Beans
- Lentils
- Pistachios
- Walnuts
- Seeds
- Cashews/Almonds

NOTES:

Mediterranean Choices Week 1

MY PREFERRED MEDITERRANEAN FOODS	NET CARBS	PROTEINS	FAT

OTHER FOODS TO EAT IN MODERATION	NET CARBS	PROTEINS	FAT

Grocery Suggestions Week 1

FRESH PRODUCE

☐ Asparagus	☐ Cauliflower	☐ Onions
☐ Avocado	☐ Celery	☐ Radishes
☐ Bell Peppers	☐ Cucumber	☐ Salad Mix
☐ Berries/Oranges/Apples/Grapes	☐ Eggplant	☐ Squash
☐ Broccoli	☐ Fennel	☐ Tomatoes
☐ Brussel Sprouts	☐ Garlic	☐ Bok Choi
☐ Cabbage	☐ Green Beans	☐ Chives
☐ Carrots	☐ Mushrooms	☐ Spinach

MEAT AND SEAFOOD

☐ Salmon	☐ Lamb	☐ Fish
☐ Tuna	☐ Beef	☐ Crab
☐ Sardines	☐ Rotisserie Chicken	☐ Lobster
☐ Oyster	☐ Turkey	☐ Scallops
☐ Shrimp	☐	☐ Mussels
☐	☐	☐

DAIRY PRODUCTS

☐ Fetta Chees	☐ Eggs	☐ Hummus
☐ Parmesan	☐ Greek Yogurt	☐ Tahini
☐ Goat Cheese	☐ Mozzarella Cheese	☐ Mayo

PANTRY ITEMS

☐ Avocado oil	☐ Tea/Coffee	☐ Tahini
☐ Dates/Figs	☐ Wholemeal Flour	☐ Sun Dried Tomatoes
☐ Bone Broth	☐ Almond Four	☐ Natural Peanut Butter
☐ Tuna, Salmon (canned)	☐ Coconut Flour	☐ Brown Sugar
☐ Cashews/Seeds	☐ Olive oil, extra virgin	☐ Almonds
☐ Coconut Oil	☐ Olives	☐ Spices
☐ Almond Milk	☐ Allowed Sweeteners	☐ Pesto

FROZEN / OTHER

☐	☐	☐
☐	☐	☐
☐	☐	☐
☐	☐	☐

Week 1 Shopping List

DATE: _____

QTY	PRODUCE

QTY	MEAT & FISH

QTY	FROZEN FOODS

QTY	DAIRY

QTY	PANTRY

QTY	OTHER/MISC.

Mediterranean Meal Plan Week 1

BREAKFAST	LUNCH	DINNER	SNACKS
BREAKFAST	LUNCH	DINNER	SNACKS
BREAKFAST	LUNCH	DINNER	SNACKS
BREAKFAST	LUNCH	DINNER	SNACKS
BREAKFAST	LUNCH	DINNER	SNACKS
BREAKFAST	LUNCH	DINNER	SNACKS
BREAKFAST	LUNCH	DINNER	SNACKS

Daily Tracker Week 1

SLEEP TRACKER:

DATE _____

RISE: _____   BEDTIME: _____   SLEEP (HRS): _____

NOTES FOR THE DAY

_____

_____

_____

EXERCISE / WORKOUT ROUTINE

TOP 6 PRIORITIES OF THE DAY

- _____   - _____
- _____   - _____
- _____   - _____

WATER INTAKE TRACKER

WATER INTAKE TRACKER

DAILY ENERGY LEVEL

HIGH	MEDIUM	LOW

BREAKFAST

FAT: CARBS: PROTEIN: CALORIES:

LUNCH

FAT: CARBS: PROTEIN: CALORIES:

DINNER

FAT: CARBS: PROTEIN: CALORIES:

SNACKS

FAT: CARBS: PROTEIN: CALORIES:

END OF THE DAY TOTAL OVERVIEW

CARBS	FAT	PROTEIN	CALORIES

Daily Tracker Week 1

SLEEP TRACKER:

DATE _____

☀ RISE: [_____]   🌙 zᶻ BEDTIME: [_____]   💭zᶻ SLEEP (HRS): [_____]

NOTES FOR THE DAY

_____
_____
_____

EXERCISE / WORKOUT ROUTINE

WATER INTAKE TRACKER

💧 💧 💧 💧 💧 💧 💧 💧

WATER INTAKE TRACKER

💧 💧 💧 💧 💧 💧 💧 💧

DAILY ENERGY LEVEL		
HIGH	MEDIUM	LOW

BREAKFAST

FAT: CARBS: PROTEIN: CALORIES:

LUNCH

FAT: CARBS: PROTEIN: CALORIES:

DINNER

FAT: CARBS: PROTEIN: CALORIES:

SNACKS

FAT: CARBS: PROTEIN: CALORIES:

TOP 6 PRIORITIES OF THE DAY

● _____   ● _____
● _____   ● _____
● _____   ● _____

END OF THE DAY TOTAL OVERVIEW

CARBS	FAT	PROTEIN	CALORIES
[____]	[____]	[____]	[____]

Daily Tracker Week 1

SLEEP TRACKER:

DATE _____

☀ RISE: _____   🌙 BEDTIME: _____   💭 SLEEP (HRS): _____

NOTES FOR THE DAY

_____
_____
_____

WATER INTAKE TRACKER

💧 💧 💧 💧 💧 💧 💧 💧

WATER INTAKE TRACKER

💧 💧 💧 💧 💧 💧 💧 💧

DAILY ENERGY LEVEL

HIGH   **MEDIUM**   **LOW**

EXERCISE / WORKOUT ROUTINE

BREAKFAST

FAT: CARBS: PROTEIN: CALORIES:

LUNCH

FAT: CARBS: PROTEIN: CALORIES:

DINNER

FAT: CARBS: PROTEIN: CALORIES:

SNACKS

FAT: CARBS: PROTEIN: CALORIES:

TOP 6 PRIORITIES OF THE DAY

- _____   - _____
- _____   - _____
- _____   - _____

END OF THE DAY TOTAL OVERVIEW

CARBS	FAT	PROTEIN	CALORIES

Daily Tracker Week 1

SLEEP TRACKER:

DATE _____

☀ RISE: [_____]   🌙 zzz BEDTIME: [_____]   💤 SLEEP (HRS): [_____]

NOTES FOR THE DAY

_____
_____
_____
_____

EXERCISE / WORKOUT ROUTINE

TOP 6 PRIORITIES OF THE DAY

- ● _____   ● _____
- ● _____   ● _____
- ● _____   ● _____

WATER INTAKE TRACKER

💧 💧 💧 💧 💧 💧 💧 💧

WATER INTAKE TRACKER

💧 💧 💧 💧 💧 💧 💧 💧

DAILY ENERGY LEVEL

HIGH	MEDIUM	LOW

BREAKFAST

FAT: CARBS: PROTEIN: CALORIES:

LUNCH

FAT: CARBS: PROTEIN: CALORIES:

DINNER

FAT: CARBS: PROTEIN: CALORIES:

SNACKS

FAT: CARBS: PROTEIN: CALORIES:

END OF THE DAY TOTAL OVERVIEW

CARBS	FAT	PROTEIN	CALORIES

Daily Tracker Week 1

SLEEP TRACKER:

DATE _____

☀ RISE: [   ]   🌙 BEDTIME: [   ]   💤 SLEEP (HRS): [   ]

NOTES FOR THE DAY

_____

_____

_____

EXERCISE / WORKOUT ROUTINE

WATER INTAKE TRACKER

💧 💧 💧 💧 💧 💧 💧 💧

WATER INTAKE TRACKER

💧 💧 💧 💧 💧 💧 💧 💧

DAILY ENERGY LEVEL

HIGH	MEDIUM	LOW

BREAKFAST

FAT: CARBS: PROTEIN: CALORIES:

LUNCH

FAT: CARBS: PROTEIN: CALORIES:

DINNER

FAT: CARBS: PROTEIN: CALORIES:

SNACKS

FAT: CARBS: PROTEIN: CALORIES:

TOP 6 PRIORITIES OF THE DAY

● _____   ● _____

● _____   ● _____

● _____   ● _____

END OF THE DAY TOTAL OVERVIEW

CARBS	FAT	PROTEIN	CALORIES
[ ]	[ ]	[ ]	[ ]

Daily Tracker Week 1

SLEEP TRACKER:

DATE _____

☀ RISE: _____   🌙 BEDTIME: _____   💭 SLEEP (HRS): _____

NOTES FOR THE DAY

_____

_____

_____

EXERCISE / WORKOUT ROUTINE

TOP 6 PRIORITIES OF THE DAY

- ⚫ _____   ⚫ _____
- ⚫ _____   ⚫ _____
- ⚫ _____   ⚫ _____

WATER INTAKE TRACKER

💧 💧 💧 💧 💧 💧 💧 💧

WATER INTAKE TRACKER

💧 💧 💧 💧 💧 💧 💧 💧

DAILY ENERGY LEVEL

HIGH	MEDIUM	LOW

BREAKFAST

FAT: CARBS: PROTEIN: CALORIES:

LUNCH

FAT: CARBS: PROTEIN: CALORIES:

DINNER

FAT: CARBS: PROTEIN: CALORIES:

SNACKS

FAT: CARBS: PROTEIN: CALORIES:

END OF THE DAY TOTAL OVERVIEW

CARBS	FAT	PROTEIN	CALORIES

Daily Tracker Week 1

SLEEP TRACKER:

DATE _____

☼ RISE: _____   🌙 BEDTIME: _____   💭 SLEEP (HRS): _____

NOTES FOR THE DAY

_____

_____

_____

EXERCISE / WORKOUT ROUTINE

TOP 6 PRIORITIES OF THE DAY

● _____   ● _____

● _____   ● _____

● _____   ● _____

WATER INTAKE TRACKER

WATER INTAKE TRACKER

DAILY ENERGY LEVEL

HIGH	MEDIUM	LOW

BREAKFAST

FAT: CARBS: PROTEIN: CALORIES:

LUNCH

FAT: CARBS: PROTEIN: CALORIES:

DINNER

FAT: CARBS: PROTEIN: CALORIES:

SNACKS

FAT: CARBS: PROTEIN: CALORIES:

END OF THE DAY TOTAL OVERVIEW

CARBS	FAT	PROTEIN	CALORIES

Week 1 Calorie Tracker

WEEK

	Breakfast	Lunch	Snacks	Dinner	Water
Monday					
	Calories	Calories	Calories	Calories	
Tuesday					
	Calories	Calories	Calories	Calories	
Wednesday					
	Calories	Calories	Calories	Calories	
Thursday					
	Calories	Calories	Calories	Calories	
Friday					
	Calories	Calories	Calories	Calories	
Saturday					
	Calories	Calories	Calories	Calories	
Sunday					
	Calories	Calories	Calories	Calories	

Week 1 Exercise Tracker

Day 1	Day 2	Day 3
Cardio ◯ Weights ◯	Cardio ◯ Weights ◯	Cardio ◯ Weights ◯

Day 4	Day 5	Day 6
Cardio ◯ Weights ◯	Cardio ◯ Weights ◯	Cardio ◯ Weights ◯

Day 7
Cardio ◯ Weights ◯

Day	Calories Burned
1	
2	
3	
4	
5	
6	
7	

Questions To Ask Yourself

Am I happy with how I did my first 7 days?

_____

_____

_____

_____

What was my biggest win?

_____

_____

_____

_____

What can I do better at?

_____

_____

_____

_____

How does my body feel?

_____

_____

_____

_____

The Mediterranean diet is perhaps the most indulgent diet of delicious foods that also keep your body healthy for years.

NOTES

Mediterranean Choices Week 2

MY PREFERRED MEDITERRANEAN FOODS	NET CARBS	PROTEINS	FAT

OTHER FOODS TO EAT IN MODERATION	NET CARBS	PROTEINS	FAT

Grocery Suggestions Week 2

FRESH PRODUCE

☐ Asparagus	☐ Cauliflower	☐ Onions
☐ Avocado	☐ Celery	☐ Radishes
☐ Bell Peppers	☐ Cucumber	☐ Salad Mix
☐ Berries/Oranges/Apples/Grapes	☐ Eggplant	☐ Squash
☐ Broccoli	☐ Fennel	☐ Tomatoes
☐ Brussel Sprouts	☐ Garlic	☐ Bok Choi
☐ Cabbage	☐ Green Beans	☐ Chives
☐ Carrots	☐ Mushrooms	☐ Spinach

MEAT AND SEAFOOD

☐ Salmon	☐ Lamb	☐ Fish
☐ Tuna	☐ Beef	☐ Crab
☐ Sardines	☐ Rotisserie Chicken	☐ Lobster
☐ Oyster	☐ Turkey	☐ Scallops
☐ Shrimp	☐	☐ Mussels
☐	☐	☐

DAIRY PRODUCTS

☐ Fetta Chees	☐ Eggs	☐ Hummus
☐ Parmesan	☐ Greek Yogurt	☐ Tahini
☐ Goat Cheese	☐ Mozzarella Cheese	☐ Mayo

PANTRY ITEMS

☐ Avocado oil	☐ Tea/Coffee	☐ Tahini
☐ Dates/Figs	☐ Wholemeal Flour	☐ Sun Dried Tomatoes
☐ Bone Broth	☐ Almond Four	☐ Natural Peanut Butter
☐ Tuna, Salmon (canned)	☐ Coconut Flour	☐ Brown Sugar
☐ Cashews/Seeds	☐ Olive oil, extra virgin	☐ Almonds
☐ Coconut Oil	☐ Olives	☐ Spices
☐ Almond Milk	☐ Allowed Sweeteners	☐ Pesto

FROZEN / OTHER

☐	☐	☐
☐	☐	☐
☐	☐	☐
☐	☐	☐

Week 2 Shopping List

DATE: _____

QTY	PRODUCE

QTY	MEAT & FISH

QTY	FROZEN FOODS

QTY	DAIRY

QTY	PANTRY

QTY	OTHER/MISC.

Mediterranean Meal Plan Week 2

BREAKFAST	LUNCH	DINNER	SNACKS
BREAKFAST	LUNCH	DINNER	SNACKS
BREAKFAST	LUNCH	DINNER	SNACKS
BREAKFAST	LUNCH	DINNER	SNACKS
BREAKFAST	LUNCH	DINNER	SNACKS
BREAKFAST	LUNCH	DINNER	SNACKS
BREAKFAST	LUNCH	DINNER	SNACKS

Daily Tracker Week 2

SLEEP TRACKER:

DATE _____

☀ RISE: _____ | 🌙 BEDTIME: _____ | 💭 SLEEP (HRS): _____

NOTES FOR THE DAY

_____
_____
_____

EXERCISE / WORKOUT ROUTINE

WATER INTAKE TRACKER

💧 💧 💧 💧 💧 💧 💧 💧

WATER INTAKE TRACKER

💧 💧 💧 💧 💧 💧 💧 💧

DAILY ENERGY LEVEL

HIGH	MEDIUM	LOW

BREAKFAST

FAT: CARBS: PROTEIN: CALORIES:

LUNCH

FAT: CARBS: PROTEIN: CALORIES:

DINNER

FAT: CARBS: PROTEIN: CALORIES:

SNACKS

FAT: CARBS: PROTEIN: CALORIES:

TOP 6 PRIORITIES OF THE DAY

● _____   ● _____
● _____   ● _____
● _____   ● _____

END OF THE DAY TOTAL OVERVIEW

CARBS	FAT	PROTEIN	CALORIES

Daily Tracker Week 2

SLEEP TRACKER:

DATE _____

☀ | RISE: | 🌙 zzz | BEDTIME: | 💭zZZ | SLEEP (HRS):

NOTES FOR THE DAY

_____

_____

_____

EXERCISE / WORKOUT ROUTINE

WATER INTAKE TRACKER

💧 💧 💧 💧 💧 💧 💧 💧

WATER INTAKE TRACKER

💧 💧 💧 💧 💧 💧 💧 💧

DAILY ENERGY LEVEL

HIGH	MEDIUM	LOW

BREAKFAST

FAT: CARBS: PROTEIN: CALORIES:

LUNCH

FAT: CARBS: PROTEIN: CALORIES:

DINNER

FAT: CARBS: PROTEIN: CALORIES:

SNACKS

FAT: CARBS: PROTEIN: CALORIES:

TOP 6 PRIORITIES OF THE DAY

- _____ - _____
- _____ - _____
- _____ - _____

END OF THE DAY TOTAL OVERVIEW

CARBS	FAT	PROTEIN	CALORIES

Daily Tracker Week 2

SLEEP TRACKER:

DATE _____

☀ RISE: [_____] 🌙 BEDTIME: [_____] 💤 SLEEP (HRS): [_____]

NOTES FOR THE DAY

_____

_____

_____

EXERCISE / WORKOUT ROUTINE

[_____]

WATER INTAKE TRACKER

💧 💧 💧 💧 💧 💧 💧 💧

WATER INTAKE TRACKER

💧 💧 💧 💧 💧 💧 💧 💧

DAILY ENERGY LEVEL

HIGH	MEDIUM	LOW

BREAKFAST

FAT: CARBS: PROTEIN: CALORIES:

LUNCH

FAT: CARBS: PROTEIN: CALORIES:

DINNER

FAT: CARBS: PROTEIN: CALORIES:

SNACKS

FAT: CARBS: PROTEIN: CALORIES:

TOP 6 PRIORITIES OF THE DAY

- _____   - _____
- _____   - _____
- _____   - _____

END OF THE DAY TOTAL OVERVIEW

CARBS	FAT	PROTEIN	CALORIES
[ ]	[ ]	[ ]	[ ]

Daily Tracker Week 2

SLEEP TRACKER:

DATE _____

☀ RISE: [_____]   🌙 BEDTIME: [_____]   💭 SLEEP (HRS): [_____]

NOTES FOR THE DAY

_____

_____

_____

EXERCISE / WORKOUT ROUTINE

WATER INTAKE TRACKER

💧 💧 💧 💧 💧 💧 💧 💧

WATER INTAKE TRACKER

💧 💧 💧 💧 💧 💧 💧 💧

DAILY ENERGY LEVEL

HIGH	MEDIUM	LOW

BREAKFAST

FAT: CARBS: PROTEIN: CALORIES:

LUNCH

FAT: CARBS: PROTEIN: CALORIES:

DINNER

FAT: CARBS: PROTEIN: CALORIES:

SNACKS

FAT: CARBS: PROTEIN: CALORIES:

TOP 6 PRIORITIES OF THE DAY

● _____   ● _____

● _____   ● _____

● _____   ● _____

END OF THE DAY TOTAL OVERVIEW

CARBS	FAT	PROTEIN	CALORIES

Daily Tracker Week 2

SLEEP TRACKER:

DATE _____

☀ RISE: _____   ☾ᶻᶻᶻ BEDTIME: _____   💭ᶻᶻᶻ SLEEP (HRS): _____

NOTES FOR THE DAY

_____

_____

_____

EXERCISE / WORKOUT ROUTINE

WATER INTAKE TRACKER

💧 💧 💧 💧 💧 💧 💧 💧

WATER INTAKE TRACKER

💧 💧 💧 💧 💧 💧 💧 💧

DAILY ENERGY LEVEL

HIGH	MEDIUM	LOW

BREAKFAST

FAT: CARBS: PROTEIN: CALORIES:

LUNCH

FAT: CARBS: PROTEIN: CALORIES:

DINNER

FAT: CARBS: PROTEIN: CALORIES:

SNACKS

FAT: CARBS: PROTEIN: CALORIES:

TOP 6 PRIORITIES OF THE DAY

● _____   ● _____

● _____   ● _____

● _____   ● _____

END OF THE DAY TOTAL OVERVIEW

CARBS	FAT	PROTEIN	CALORIES

Daily Tracker Week 2

SLEEP TRACKER:

DATE _____

☀ RISE: [   ]   🌙 BEDTIME: [   ]   💤 SLEEP (HRS): [   ]

NOTES FOR THE DAY

_____
_____
_____

EXERCISE / WORKOUT ROUTINE

WATER INTAKE TRACKER

💧 💧 💧 💧 💧 💧 💧 💧

WATER INTAKE TRACKER

💧 💧 💧 💧 💧 💧 💧 💧

DAILY ENERGY LEVEL

HIGH	MEDIUM	LOW

BREAKFAST

FAT: CARBS: PROTEIN: CALORIES:

LUNCH

FAT: CARBS: PROTEIN: CALORIES:

DINNER

FAT: CARBS: PROTEIN: CALORIES:

SNACKS

FAT: CARBS: PROTEIN: CALORIES:

TOP 6 PRIORITIES OF THE DAY

● _____   ● _____

● _____   ● _____

● _____   ● _____

END OF THE DAY TOTAL OVERVIEW

CARBS	FAT	PROTEIN	CALORIES
[ ]	[ ]	[ ]	[ ]

Daily Tracker Week 2

SLEEP TRACKER:

DATE _____

☀ RISE: [ ]   🌙 BEDTIME: [ ]   💭 SLEEP (HRS): [ ]

NOTES FOR THE DAY

_____

_____

_____

EXERCISE / WORKOUT ROUTINE

WATER INTAKE TRACKER

WATER INTAKE TRACKER

DAILY ENERGY LEVEL

HIGH	MEDIUM	LOW

BREAKFAST

FAT: CARBS: PROTEIN: CALORIES:

LUNCH

FAT: CARBS: PROTEIN: CALORIES:

DINNER

FAT: CARBS: PROTEIN: CALORIES:

SNACKS

FAT: CARBS: PROTEIN: CALORIES:

TOP 6 PRIORITIES OF THE DAY

- _____ - _____
- _____ - _____
- _____ - _____

END OF THE DAY TOTAL OVERVIEW

CARBS	FAT	PROTEIN	CALORIES
[ ]	[ ]	[ ]	[ ]

Week 2 Calorie Tracker

WEEK

	Breakfast	Lunch	Snacks	Dinner	Water
Monday					
	Calories	Calories	Calories	Calories	
Tuesday					
	Calories	Calories	Calories	Calories	
Wednesday					
	Calories	Calories	Calories	Calories	
Thursday					
	Calories	Calories	Calories	Calories	
Friday					
	Calories	Calories	Calories	Calories	
Saturday					
	Calories	Calories	Calories	Calories	
Sunday					
	Calories	Calories	Calories	Calories	

Week 2Exercise Tracker

Day 1	Day 2	Day 3
Cardio ○ Weights ○	Cardio ○ Weights ○	Cardio ○ Weights ○

Day 4	Day 5	Day 6
Cardio ○ Weights ○	Cardio ○ Weights ○	Cardio ○ Weights ○

Day 7	Day	Calories Burned
	1	
	2	
	3	
	4	
	5	
Cardio ○	6	
Weights○	7	

Questions To Ask Yourself

Am I happy with how I did my first 14 days?

_____

_____

_____

_____

What was my biggest win?

_____

_____

_____

_____

What can I do better at?

_____

_____

_____

_____

How does my body feel?

_____

_____

_____

_____

Eat is if you're traveling to the Mediterranean Sea and enjoying all of the fresh cuisine the surrounding countries have to offer

NOTES

Mediterranean Choices Week 3

MY PREFERRED MEDITERRANEAN FOODS	NET CARBS	PROTEINS	FAT

OTHER FOODS TO EAT IN MODERATION	NET CARBS	PROTEINS	FAT

Grocery Suggestions Week 3

FRESH PRODUCE

☐ Asparagus	☐ Cauliflower	☐ Onions
☐ Avocado	☐ Celery	☐ Radishes
☐ Bell Peppers	☐ Cucumber	☐ Salad Mix
☐ Berries/Oranges/Apples/Grapes	☐ Eggplant	☐ Squash
☐ Broccoli	☐ Fennel	☐ Tomatoes
☐ Brussel Sprouts	☐ Garlic	☐ Bok Choi
☐ Cabbage	☐ Green Beans	☐ Chives
☐ Carrots	☐ Mushrooms	☐ Spinach

MEAT AND SEAFOOD

☐ Salmon	☐ Lamb	☐ Fish
☐ Tuna	☐ Beef	☐ Crab
☐ Sardines	☐ Rotisserie Chicken	☐ Lobster
☐ Oyster	☐ Turkey	☐ Scallops
☐ Shrimp	☐	☐ Mussels
☐	☐	☐

DAIRY PRODUCTS

☐ Fetta Chees	☐ Eggs	☐ Hummus
☐ Parmesan	☐ Greek Yogurt	☐ Tahini
☐ Goat Cheese	☐ Mozzarella Cheese	☐ Mayo

PANTRY ITEMS

☐ Avocado oil	☐ Tea/Coffee	☐ Tahini
☐ Dates/Figs	☐ Wholemeal Flour	☐ Sun Dried Tomatoes
☐ Bone Broth	☐ Almond Four	☐ Natural Peanut Butter
☐ Tuna, Salmon (canned)	☐ Coconut Flour	☐ Brown Sugar
☐ Cashews/Seeds	☐ Olive oil, extra virgin	☐ Almonds
☐ Coconut Oil	☐ Olives	☐ Spices
☐ Almond Milk	☐ Allowed Sweeteners	☐ Pesto

FROZEN / OTHER

☐	☐	☐
☐	☐	☐
☐	☐	☐

Week 3 Shopping List

DATE: _____

QTY	PRODUCE

QTY	MEAT & FISH

QTY	FROZEN FOODS

QTY	DAIRY

QTY	PANTRY

QTY	OTHER/MISC.

Mediterranean Meal Plan Week 3

BREAKFAST	LUNCH	DINNER	SNACKS
BREAKFAST	LUNCH	DINNER	SNACKS
BREAKFAST	LUNCH	DINNER	SNACKS
BREAKFAST	LUNCH	DINNER	SNACKS
BREAKFAST	LUNCH	DINNER	SNACKS
BREAKFAST	LUNCH	DINNER	SNACKS
BREAKFAST	LUNCH	DINNER	SNACKS

Daily Tracker Week 3

SLEEP TRACKER:

DATE _____

☀ RISE: _____　🌙 BEDTIME: _____　💭 SLEEP (HRS): _____

NOTES FOR THE DAY

_____

_____

_____

EXERCISE / WORKOUT ROUTINE

TOP 6 PRIORITIES OF THE DAY

- ● _____
- ● _____
- ● _____
- ● _____
- ● _____
- ● _____

WATER INTAKE TRACKER

💧 💧 💧 💧 💧 💧 💧 💧

WATER INTAKE TRACKER

💧 💧 💧 💧 💧 💧 💧 💧

DAILY ENERGY LEVEL

HIGH	MEDIUM	LOW

BREAKFAST

FAT:　　CARBS:　　PROTEIN:　　CALORIES:

LUNCH

FAT:　　CARBS:　　PROTEIN:　　CALORIES:

DINNER

FAT:　　CARBS:　　PROTEIN:　　CALORIES:

SNACKS

FAT:　　CARBS:　　PROTEIN:　　CALORIES:

END OF THE DAY TOTAL OVERVIEW

CARBS	FAT	PROTEIN	CALORIES

Daily Tracker Week 3

SLEEP TRACKER:

DATE _____

☀ RISE: _____   🌙 BEDTIME: _____   💤 SLEEP (HRS): _____

NOTES FOR THE DAY

_____
_____
_____

EXERCISE / WORKOUT ROUTINE

TOP 6 PRIORITIES OF THE DAY

- _____   - _____
- _____   - _____
- _____   - _____

WATER INTAKE TRACKER

WATER INTAKE TRACKER

DAILY ENERGY LEVEL

HIGH	MEDIUM	LOW

BREAKFAST

FAT: CARBS: PROTEIN: CALORIES:

LUNCH

FAT: CARBS: PROTEIN: CALORIES:

DINNER

FAT: CARBS: PROTEIN: CALORIES:

SNACKS

FAT: CARBS: PROTEIN: CALORIES:

END OF THE DAY TOTAL OVERVIEW

CARBS	FAT	PROTEIN	CALORIES

Daily Tracker Week 3

SLEEP TRACKER:

DATE _____

☀ RISE: [   ]   🌙 BEDTIME: [   ]   💭 SLEEP (HRS): [   ]

NOTES FOR THE DAY

_____

_____

_____

EXERCISE / WORKOUT ROUTINE

TOP 6 PRIORITIES OF THE DAY

● _____   ● _____

● _____   ● _____

● _____   ● _____

WATER INTAKE TRACKER

💧 💧 💧 💧 💧 💧 💧 💧

WATER INTAKE TRACKER

💧 💧 💧 💧 💧 💧 💧 💧

DAILY ENERGY LEVEL

HIGH	**MEDIUM**	**LOW**

BREAKFAST

FAT: CARBS: PROTEIN: CALORIES:

LUNCH

FAT: CARBS: PROTEIN: CALORIES:

DINNER

FAT: CARBS: PROTEIN: CALORIES:

SNACKS

FAT: CARBS: PROTEIN: CALORIES:

END OF THE DAY TOTAL OVERVIEW

CARBS	FAT	PROTEIN	CALORIES
[ ]	[ ]	[ ]	[ ]

Daily Tracker Week 3

SLEEP TRACKER:

DATE _____

☼ RISE: _____ 🌙 BEDTIME: _____ 💤 SLEEP (HRS): _____

NOTES FOR THE DAY

_____
_____
_____

EXERCISE / WORKOUT ROUTINE

TOP 6 PRIORITIES OF THE DAY

- • _____
- • _____
- • _____

- • _____
- • _____
- • _____

WATER INTAKE TRACKER

WATER INTAKE TRACKER

DAILY ENERGY LEVEL

HIGH	MEDIUM	LOW

BREAKFAST

FAT:	CARBS:	PROTEIN:	CALORIES:

LUNCH

FAT:	CARBS:	PROTEIN:	CALORIES:

DINNER

FAT:	CARBS:	PROTEIN:	CALORIES:

SNACKS

FAT:	CARBS:	PROTEIN:	CALORIES:

END OF THE DAY TOTAL OVERVIEW

CARBS	FAT	PROTEIN	CALORIES

Daily Tracker Week 3

SLEEP TRACKER:

DATE _____

☀ RISE: | 🌙 BEDTIME: | 💤 SLEEP (HRS):

NOTES FOR THE DAY

_____

_____

_____

EXERCISE / WORKOUT ROUTINE

WATER INTAKE TRACKER

💧 💧 💧 💧 💧 💧 💧 💧

WATER INTAKE TRACKER

💧 💧 💧 💧 💧 💧 💧 💧

DAILY ENERGY LEVEL

HIGH	MEDIUM	LOW

BREAKFAST

FAT: | CARBS: | PROTEIN: | CALORIES:

LUNCH

FAT: | CARBS: | PROTEIN: | CALORIES:

DINNER

FAT: | CARBS: | PROTEIN: | CALORIES:

SNACKS

FAT: | CARBS: | PROTEIN: | CALORIES:

TOP 6 PRIORITIES OF THE DAY

- _____ - _____
- _____ - _____
- _____ - _____

END OF THE DAY TOTAL OVERVIEW

CARBS	FAT	PROTEIN	CALORIES

Daily Tracker Week 3

SLEEP TRACKER:

DATE _____

RISE: [   ]   BEDTIME: [   ]   SLEEP (HRS): [   ]

NOTES FOR THE DAY

_____

_____

_____

EXERCISE / WORKOUT ROUTINE

WATER INTAKE TRACKER

WATER INTAKE TRACKER

DAILY ENERGY LEVEL

HIGH	MEDIUM	LOW

BREAKFAST

FAT: CARBS: PROTEIN: CALORIES:

LUNCH

FAT: CARBS: PROTEIN: CALORIES:

DINNER

FAT: CARBS: PROTEIN: CALORIES:

SNACKS

FAT: CARBS: PROTEIN: CALORIES:

TOP 6 PRIORITIES OF THE DAY

- _____   - _____
- _____   - _____
- _____   - _____

END OF THE DAY TOTAL OVERVIEW

CARBS	FAT	PROTEIN	CALORIES

Daily Tracker Week 3

SLEEP TRACKER:

DATE _____

☀ RISE: [   ]   🌙 BEDTIME: [   ]   💭 SLEEP (HRS): [   ]

NOTES FOR THE DAY

_____

_____

_____

EXERCISE / WORKOUT ROUTINE

WATER INTAKE TRACKER

💧 💧 💧 💧 💧 💧 💧 💧

WATER INTAKE TRACKER

💧 💧 💧 💧 💧 💧 💧 💧

DAILY ENERGY LEVEL

HIGH	MEDIUM	LOW

BREAKFAST

FAT: CARBS: PROTEIN: CALORIES:

LUNCH

FAT: CARBS: PROTEIN: CALORIES:

DINNER

FAT: CARBS: PROTEIN: CALORIES:

SNACKS

FAT: CARBS: PROTEIN: CALORIES:

TOP 6 PRIORITIES OF THE DAY

● _____   ● _____

● _____   ● _____

● _____   ● _____

END OF THE DAY TOTAL OVERVIEW

CARBS	FAT	PROTEIN	CALORIES
[ ]	[ ]	[ ]	[ ]

Week 3 Calorie Tracker

WEEK

	Breakfast	Lunch	Snacks	Dinner	Water
Monday					
	Calories	Calories	Calories	Calories	
Tuesday					
	Calories	Calories	Calories	Calories	
Wednesday					
	Calories	Calories	Calories	Calories	
Thursday					
	Calories	Calories	Calories	Calories	
Friday					
	Calories	Calories	Calories	Calories	
Saturday					
	Calories	Calories	Calories	Calories	
Sunday					
	Calories	Calories	Calories	Calories	

Week 3 Exercise Tracker

Day 1	Day 2	Day 3
Cardio ○ Weights ○	Cardio ○ Weights ○	Cardio ○ Weights ○

Day 4	Day 5	Day 6
Cardio ○ Weights ○	Cardio ○ Weights ○	Cardio ○ Weights ○

Day 7		Day	Calories Burned
		1	
		2	
		3	
		4	
		5	
Cardio ○		6	
Weights ○		7	

Questions To Ask Yourself

Am I happy with how I did my first 21 days?

_____

_____

_____

_____

What was my biggest win?

_____

_____

_____

_____

What can I do better at?

_____

_____

_____

_____

How does my body feel?

_____

_____

_____

_____

Enjoy fresh meats, vegetables, fruits, nuts, healthy fat – and even wine on this diet, without giving it a second thought.

NOTES

Mediterranean Choices Week 4

MY PREFERRED MEDITERRANEAN FOODS	NET CARBS	PROTEINS	FAT

OTHER FOODS TO EAT IN MODERATION	NET CARBS	PROTEINS	FAT

Daily Tracker Week 4

DATE _____

RISE: _____   BEDTIME: _____   SLEEP (HRS): _____

NOTES FOR THE DAY

_____

_____

_____

WATER INTAKE TRACKER

WATER INTAKE TRACKER

EXERCISE / WORKOUT ROUTINE

DAILY ENERGY LEVEL

HIGH	MEDIUM	LOW

BREAKFAST

FAT: CARBS: PROTEIN: CALORIES:

LUNCH

FAT: CARBS: PROTEIN: CALORIES:

DINNER

FAT: CARBS: PROTEIN: CALORIES:

SNACKS

FAT: CARBS: PROTEIN: CALORIES:

TOP 6 PRIORITIES OF THE DAY

- _____   - _____
- _____   - _____
- _____   - _____

END OF THE DAY TOTAL OVERVIEW

CARBS	FAT	PROTEIN	CALORIES

Daily Tracker Week 4

SLEEP TRACKER:

DATE _____

☼ RISE: | 🌙 BEDTIME: | 💭 SLEEP (HRS):

NOTES FOR THE DAY

WATER INTAKE TRACKER

💧 💧 💧 💧 💧 💧 💧 💧

WATER INTAKE TRACKER

💧 💧 💧 💧 💧 💧 💧 💧

EXERCISE / WORKOUT ROUTINE

DAILY ENERGY LEVEL

HIGH	MEDIUM	LOW

BREAKFAST

FAT: | CARBS: | PROTEIN: | CALORIES:

LUNCH

FAT: | CARBS: | PROTEIN: | CALORIES:

DINNER

FAT: | CARBS: | PROTEIN: | CALORIES:

SNACKS

FAT: | CARBS: | PROTEIN: | CALORIES:

TOP 6 PRIORITIES OF THE DAY

-
-
-
-
-
-

END OF THE DAY TOTAL OVERVIEW

CARBS	FAT	PROTEIN	CALORIES

Daily Tracker Week 4

SLEEP TRACKER:

DATE _____

☀ RISE: [   ]   🌙 BEDTIME: [   ]   💤 SLEEP (HRS): [   ]

NOTES FOR THE DAY

_____

_____

_____

EXERCISE / WORKOUT ROUTINE

TOP 6 PRIORITIES OF THE DAY

● _____   ● _____

● _____   ● _____

● _____   ● _____

WATER INTAKE TRACKER

💧 💧 💧 💧 💧 💧 💧 💧

WATER INTAKE TRACKER

💧 💧 💧 💧 💧 💧 💧 💧

DAILY ENERGY LEVEL

HIGH   **MEDIUM**   **LOW**

BREAKFAST

FAT: CARBS: PROTEIN: CALORIES:

LUNCH

FAT: CARBS: PROTEIN: CALORIES:

DINNER

FAT: CARBS: PROTEIN: CALORIES:

SNACKS

FAT: CARBS: PROTEIN: CALORIES:

END OF THE DAY TOTAL OVERVIEW

CARBS   FAT   PROTEIN   CALORIES

_____   _____   _____   _____

[   ]   [   ]   [   ]   [   ]

Daily Tracker Week 4

SLEEP TRACKER:

DATE _____

☼ RISE: _____   🌙 BEDTIME: _____   💭 SLEEP (HRS): _____

NOTES FOR THE DAY

_____
_____
_____

EXERCISE / WORKOUT ROUTINE

TOP 6 PRIORITIES OF THE DAY

• _____   • _____
• _____   • _____
• _____   • _____

WATER INTAKE TRACKER

WATER INTAKE TRACKER

DAILY ENERGY LEVEL

HIGH	MEDIUM	LOW

BREAKFAST

FAT: CARBS: PROTEIN: CALORIES:

LUNCH

FAT: CARBS: PROTEIN: CALORIES:

DINNER

FAT: CARBS: PROTEIN: CALORIES:

SNACKS

FAT: CARBS: PROTEIN: CALORIES:

END OF THE DAY TOTAL OVERVIEW

CARBS	FAT	PROTEIN	CALORIES

Daily Tracker Week 4

SLEEP TRACKER:

DATE _____

RISE: | BEDTIME: | SLEEP (HRS):

NOTES FOR THE DAY

_____

_____

_____

EXERCISE / WORKOUT ROUTINE

WATER INTAKE TRACKER

WATER INTAKE TRACKER

DAILY ENERGY LEVEL

| HIGH | MEDIUM | LOW |

BREAKFAST

FAT: | CARBS: | PROTEIN: | CALORIES:

LUNCH

FAT: | CARBS: | PROTEIN: | CALORIES:

DINNER

FAT: | CARBS: | PROTEIN: | CALORIES:

SNACKS

FAT: | CARBS: | PROTEIN: | CALORIES:

TOP 6 PRIORITIES OF THE DAY

END OF THE DAY TOTAL OVERVIEW

| CARBS | FAT | PROTEIN | CALORIES |

Daily Tracker Week 4

SLEEP TRACKER:

DATE _____

RISE: | BEDTIME: | SLEEP (HRS):

NOTES FOR THE DAY

_____
_____
_____
_____

WATER INTAKE TRACKER

WATER INTAKE TRACKER

EXERCISE / WORKOUT ROUTINE

DAILY ENERGY LEVEL

HIGH	MEDIUM	LOW

BREAKFAST

FAT: | CARBS: | PROTEIN: | CALORIES:

LUNCH

FAT: | CARBS: | PROTEIN: | CALORIES:

DINNER

FAT: | CARBS: | PROTEIN: | CALORIES:

SNACKS

FAT: | CARBS: | PROTEIN: | CALORIES:

TOP 6 PRIORITIES OF THE DAY

-
-
-
-
-
-

END OF THE DAY TOTAL OVERVIEW

CARBS | FAT | PROTEIN | CALORIES

Daily Tracker Week 4

SLEEP TRACKER:

DATE _____

☀ RISE: _____ 🌙 zᶻᶻ BEDTIME: _____ 💭 zᶻᶻ SLEEP (HRS): _____

NOTES FOR THE DAY

_____

_____

_____

EXERCISE / WORKOUT ROUTINE

TOP 6 PRIORITIES OF THE DAY

● _____ ● _____

● _____ ● _____

● _____ ● _____

WATER INTAKE TRACKER

💧 💧 💧 💧 💧 💧 💧 💧

WATER INTAKE TRACKER

💧 💧 💧 💧 💧 💧 💧 💧

DAILY ENERGY LEVEL

HIGH	MEDIUM	LOW

BREAKFAST

FAT: CARBS: PROTEIN: CALORIES:

LUNCH

FAT: CARBS: PROTEIN: CALORIES:

DINNER

FAT: CARBS: PROTEIN: CALORIES:

SNACKS

FAT: CARBS: PROTEIN: CALORIES:

END OF THE DAY TOTAL OVERVIEW

CARBS	FAT	PROTEIN	CALORIES

Grocery Suggestions Week 4

FRESH PRODUCE

☐ Asparagus	☐ Cauliflower	☐ Onions
☐ Avocado	☐ Celery	☐ Radishes
☐ Bell Peppers	☐ Cucumber	☐ Salad Mix
☐ Berries/Oranges/Apples/Grapes	☐ Eggplant	☐ Squash
☐ Broccoli	☐ Fennel	☐ Tomatoes
☐ Brussel Sprouts	☐ Garlic	☐ Bok Choi
☐ Cabbage	☐ Green Beans	☐ Chives
☐ Carrots	☐ Mushrooms	☐ Spinach

MEAT AND SEAFOOD

☐ Salmon	☐ Lamb	☐ Fish
☐ Tuna	☐ Beef	☐ Crab
☐ Sardines	☐ Rotisserie Chicken	☐ Lobster
☐ Oyster	☐ Turkey	☐ Scallops
☐ Shrimp	☐	☐ Mussels
☐	☐	☐

DAIRY PRODUCTS

☐ Fetta Chees	☐ Eggs	☐ Hummus
☐ Parmesan	☐ Greek Yogurt	☐ Tahini
☐ Goat Cheese	☐ Mozzarella Cheese	☐ Mayo

PANTRY ITEMS

☐ Avocado oil	☐ Tea/Coffee	☐ Tahini
☐ Dates/Figs	☐ Wholemeal Flour	☐ Sun Dried Tomatoes
☐ Bone Broth	☐ Almond Four	☐ Natural Peanut Butter
☐ Tuna, Salmon (canned)	☐ Coconut Flour	☐ Brown Sugar
☐ Cashews/Seeds	☐ Olive oil, extra virgin	☐ Almonds
☐ Coconut Oil	☐ Olives	☐ Spices
☐ Almond Milk	☐ Allowed Sweeteners	☐ Pesto

FROZEN / OTHER

☐	☐	☐
☐	☐	☐
☐	☐	☐
☐	☐	☐

Week 4 Shopping List

DATE: _____

QTY	PRODUCE

QTY	MEAT & FISH

QTY	FROZEN FOODS

QTY	DAIRY

QTY	PANTRY

QTY	OTHER/MISC.

Mediterranean Meal Plan Week 4

BREAKFAST	LUNCH	DINNER	SNACKS

BREAKFAST	LUNCH	DINNER	SNACKS

BREAKFAST	LUNCH	DINNER	SNACKS

BREAKFAST	LUNCH	DINNER	SNACKS

BREAKFAST	LUNCH	DINNER	SNACKS

BREAKFAST	LUNCH	DINNER	SNACKS

BREAKFAST	LUNCH	DINNER	SNACKS

Week 4 Calorie Tracker

WEEK

	Breakfast	Lunch	Snacks	Dinner	Water
Monday					
	Calories	Calories	Calories	Calories	
Tuesday					
	Calories	Calories	Calories	Calories	
Wednesday					
	Calories	Calories	Calories	Calories	
Thursday					
	Calories	Calories	Calories	Calories	
Friday					
	Calories	Calories	Calories	Calories	
Saturday					
	Calories	Calories	Calories	Calories	
Sunday					
	Calories	Calories	Calories	Calories	

Week 4 Exercise Tracker

Day 1	Day 2	Day 3
Cardio ○ Weights ○	Cardio ○ Weights ○	Cardio ○ Weights ○

Day 4	Day 5	Day 6
Cardio ○ Weights ○	Cardio ○ Weights ○	Cardio ○ Weights ○

Day 7		Day	Calories Burned
		1	
		2	
		3	
		4	
		5	
Cardio ○		6	
Weights ○		7	

Questions To Ask Yourself

Am I happy with how I did my first 28 days?

_____

_____

_____

_____

What was my biggest win?

_____

_____

_____

_____

What can I do better at?

_____

_____

_____

_____

How does my body feel?

_____

_____

_____

_____

The Mediterranean Diet helps stabilize your blood sugar throughout the day

NOTES

Favorite Recipes

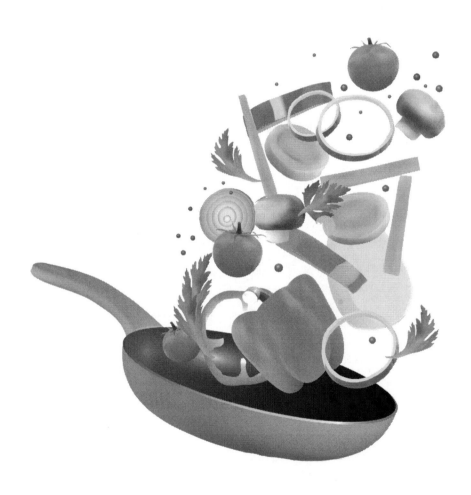

Mediterranean Recipe

RECIPE NAME:

Mediterranean	Low Carb	Paleo	Vegetarian	Vegan	Dairy Free	Gluten Free
☐	☐	☐	☐	☐	☐	☐

QTY	INGREDIENTS	RECIPE INSTRUCTIONS

NOTES & RECIPE REVIEW

Serves	
Prep Time	
Cook Time	
Tools	
Temp	

Total	Carbs	Fat	Protein	Cals

Mediterranean *Recipe*

RECIPE NAME:

	Mediterranean	Low Carb	Paleo	Vegetarian	Vegan	Dairy Free	Gluten Free
	☐	☐	☐	☐	☐	☐	☐

QTY	INGREDIENTS	RECIPE INSTRUCTIONS

NOTES & RECIPE REVIEW	
	Serves
	Prep Time
	Cook Time
	Tools
	Temp

Total	Carbs	Fat	Protein	Cals

Mediterranean *Recipe*

RECIPE NAME:

	Mediterranean	Low Carb	Paleo	Vegetarian	Vegan	Dairy Free	Gluten Free
	☐	☐	☐	☐	☐	☐	☐

QTY	INGREDIENTS	RECIPE INSTRUCTIONS

NOTES & RECIPE REVIEW

Serves	
Prep Time	
Cook Time	
Tools	
Temp	

Total	Carbs	Fat	Protein	Cals

Mediterranean *Recipe*

RECIPE NAME:

	Mediterranean	Low Carb	Paleo	Vegetarian	Vegan	Dairy Free	Gluten Free
	☐	☐	☐	☐	☐	☐	☐

QTY	INGREDIENTS

RECIPE INSTRUCTIONS

NOTES & RECIPE REVIEW

Serves	
Prep Time	
Cook Time	
Tools	
Temp	

Total	Carbs	Fat	Protein	Cals

Mediterranean *Recipe*

RECIPE NAME:

	Mediterranean	Low Carb	Paleo	Vegetarian	Vegan	Dairy Free	Gluten Free
	☐	☐	☐	☐	☐	☐	☐

QTY	INGREDIENTS

RECIPE INSTRUCTIONS

NOTES & RECIPE REVIEW

Serves	
Prep Time	
Cook Time	
Tools	
Temp	

Total	Carbs	Fat	Protein	Cals

Mediterranean *Recipe*

RECIPE NAME:

Mediterranean	Low Carb	Paleo	Vegetarian	Vegan	Dairy Free	Gluten Free
☐	☐	☐	☐	☐	☐	☐

QTY	INGREDIENTS

RECIPE INSTRUCTIONS

NOTES & RECIPE REVIEW

Serves	
Prep Time	
Cook Time	
Tools	
Temp	

Total	Carbs	Fat	Protein	Cals

Mediterranean *Recipe*

RECIPE NAME:

	Mediterranean	Low Carb	Paleo	Vegetarian	Vegan	Dairy Free	Gluten Free
	☐	☐	☐	☐	☐	☐	☐

QTY	INGREDIENTS

RECIPE INSTRUCTIONS

NOTES & RECIPE REVIEW

Serves	
Prep Time	
Cook Time	
Tools	
Temp	

Total	Carbs	Fat	Protein	Cals

Mediterranean *Recipe*

RECIPE NAME:

	Mediterranean	Low Carb	Paleo	Vegetarian	Vegan	Dairy Free	Gluten Free
	☐	☐	☐	☐	☐	☐	☐

QTY	INGREDIENTS

RECIPE INSTRUCTIONS

NOTES & RECIPE REVIEW

Serves	
Prep Time	
Cook Time	
Tools	
Temp	

Total	Carbs	Fat	Protein	Cals

Mediterranean *Recipe*

RECIPE NAME:

Mediterranean	Low Carb	Paleo	Vegetarian	Vegan	Dairy Free	Gluten Free
☐	☐	☐	☐	☐	☐	☐

QTY	INGREDIENTS	RECIPE INSTRUCTIONS

NOTES & RECIPE REVIEW

Serves	
Prep Time	
Cook Time	
Tools	
Temp	

Total	Carbs	Fat	Protein	Cals

Mediterranean *Recipe*

RECIPE NAME:

	Mediterranean	Low Carb	Paleo	Vegetarian	Vegan	Dairy Free	Gluten Free
	☐	☐	☐	☐	☐	☐	☐

QTY	INGREDIENTS	RECIPE INSTRUCTIONS

NOTES & RECIPE REVIEW

Serves	
Prep Time	
Cook Time	
Tools	
Temp	

Total	Carbs	Fat	Protein	Cals

Mediterranean *Recipe*

RECIPE NAME:

	Mediterrane an	Low Carb	Paleo	Vegetarian	Vegan	Dairy Free	Gluten Free
	☐	☐	☐	☐	☐	☐	☐

QTY	INGREDIENTS	RECIPE INSTRUCTIONS

NOTES & RECIPE REVIEW

Serves	
Prep Time	
Cook Time	
Tools	
Temp	

Total	Carbs	Fat	Protein	Cals

Mediterranean *Recipe*

RECIPE NAME:

Mediterranean	Low Carb	Paleo	Vegetarian	Vegan	Dairy Free	Gluten Free
☐	☐	☐	☐	☐	☐	☐

QTY	INGREDIENTS

RECIPE INSTRUCTIONS

NOTES & RECIPE REVIEW

Serves	
Prep Time	
Cook Time	
Tools	
Temp	

Total	Carbs	Fat	Protein	Cals

Mediterranean *Recipe*

RECIPE NAME:

	Mediterranean	Low Carb	Paleo	Vegetarian	Vegan	Dairy Free	Gluten Free
	☐	☐	☐	☐	☐	☐	☐

QTY	INGREDIENTS	RECIPE INSTRUCTIONS

NOTES & RECIPE REVIEW		
	Serves	
	Prep Time	
	Cook Time	
	Tools	
	Temp	

Total	Carbs	Fat	Protein	Cals

Mediterranean *Recipe*

RECIPE NAME:

	Mediterranean	Low Carb	Paleo	Vegetarian	Vegan	Dairy Free	Gluten Free
	☐	☐	☐	☐	☐	☐	☐

QTY	INGREDIENTS

RECIPE INSTRUCTIONS

NOTES & RECIPE REVIEW

Serves	
Prep Time	
Cook Time	
Tools	
Temp	

Total	Carbs	Fat	Protein	Cals

Mediterranean *Recipe*

RECIPE NAME:

Mediterranean	Low Carb	Paleo	Vegetarian	Vegan	Dairy Free	Gluten Free
☐	☐	☐	☐	☐	☐	☐

QTY	INGREDIENTS

RECIPE INSTRUCTIONS

NOTES & RECIPE REVIEW

Serves	
Prep Time	
Cook Time	
Tools	
Temp	

Total	Carbs	Fat	Protein	Cals

Mediterranean *Recipe*

RECIPE NAME:

	Mediterranean	Low Carb	Paleo	Vegetarian	Vegan	Dairy Free	Gluten Free
	☐	☐	☐	☐	☐	☐	☐

QTY	INGREDIENTS	RECIPE INSTRUCTIONS

NOTES & RECIPE REVIEW		
	Serves	
	Prep Time	
	Cook Time	
	Tools	
	Temp	

Total	Carbs	Fat	Protein	Cals

Mediterranean *Recipe*

RECIPE NAME:

	Mediterranean	Low Carb	Paleo	Vegetarian	Vegan	Dairy Free	Gluten Free
	☐	☐	☐	☐	☐	☐	☐

QTY	INGREDIENTS

RECIPE INSTRUCTIONS

NOTES & RECIPE REVIEW

Serves	
Prep Time	
Cook Time	
Tools	
Temp	

Total	Carbs	Fat	Protein	Cals

Mediterranean *Recipe*

RECIPE NAME:

	Mediterranean	Low Carb	Paleo	Vegetarian	Vegan	Dairy Free	Gluten Free
	☐	☐	☐	☐	☐	☐	☐

QTY	INGREDIENTS

RECIPE INSTRUCTIONS

NOTES & RECIPE REVIEW

Serves	
Prep Time	
Cook Time	
Tools	
Temp	

Total	Carbs	Fat	Protein	Cals

Mediterranean *Recipe*

RECIPE NAME:

Mediterranean	Low Carb	Paleo	Vegetarian	Vegan	Dairy Free	Gluten Free
☐	☐	☐	☐	☐	☐	☐

QTY	INGREDIENTS	RECIPE INSTRUCTIONS

NOTES & RECIPE REVIEW

Serves	
Prep Time	
Cook Time	
Tools	
Temp	

Total	Carbs	Fat	Protein	Cals

Mediterranean *Recipe*

RECIPE NAME:

Mediterranean	Low Carb	Paleo	Vegetarian	Vegan	Dairy Free	Gluten Free
☐	☐	☐	☐	☐	☐	☐

QTY	INGREDIENTS	RECIPE INSTRUCTIONS

NOTES & RECIPE REVIEW

Serves	
Prep Time	
Cook Time	
Tools	
Temp	

Total	Carbs	Fat	Protein	Cals

Mediterranean Recipe

RECIPE NAME:

_____

	Mediterranean	Low Carb	Paleo	Vegetarian	Vegan	Dairy Free	Gluten Free
	☐	☐	☐	☐	☐	☐	☐

QTY	INGREDIENTS	RECIPE INSTRUCTIONS

NOTES & RECIPE REVIEW		
	Serves	
	Prep Time	
	Cook Time	
	Tools	
	Temp	

Total	Carbs	Fat	Protein	Cals

Mediterranean *Recipe*

RECIPE NAME:

	Mediterranean	Low Carb	Paleo	Vegetarian	Vegan	Dairy Free	Gluten Free
	☐	☐	☐	☐	☐	☐	☐

QTY	INGREDIENTS

RECIPE INSTRUCTIONS

NOTES & RECIPE REVIEW

Serves	
Prep Time	
Cook Time	
Tools	
Temp	

Total	Carbs	Fat	Protein	Cals

Mediterranean *Recipe*

RECIPE NAME:

	Mediterranean	Low Carb	Paleo	Vegetarian	Vegan	Dairy Free	Gluten Free
	☐	☐	☐	☐	☐	☐	☐

QTY	INGREDIENTS	RECIPE INSTRUCTIONS

NOTES & RECIPE REVIEW

Serves	
Prep Time	
Cook Time	
Tools	
Temp	

Total	Carbs	Fat	Protein	Cals

Mediterranean *Recipe*

RECIPE NAME:

	Mediterranean	Low Carb	Paleo	Vegetarian	Vegan	Dairy Free	Gluten Free
	☐	☐	☐	☐	☐	☐	☐

QTY	INGREDIENTS	RECIPE INSTRUCTIONS

NOTES & RECIPE REVIEW

Serves	
Prep Time	
Cook Time	
Tools	
Temp	

Total	Carbs	Fat	Protein	Cals

Mediterranean *Recipe*

RECIPE NAME:

	Mediterranean	Low Carb	Paleo	Vegetarian	Vegan	Dairy Free	Gluten Free
	☐	☐	☐	☐	☐	☐	☐

QTY	INGREDIENTS	RECIPE INSTRUCTIONS

NOTES & RECIPE REVIEW		
	Serves	
	Prep Time	
	Cook Time	
	Tools	
	Temp	

Total	Carbs	Fat	Protein	Cals

Mediterranean *Recipe*

RECIPE NAME:

_____

Mediterranean	Low Carb	Paleo	Vegetarian	Vegan	Dairy Free	Gluten Free
☐	☐	☐	☐	☐	☐	☐

QTY	INGREDIENTS	RECIPE INSTRUCTIONS

NOTES & RECIPE REVIEW

	Serves
	Prep Time
	Cook Time
	Tools
	Temp

Total	Carbs	Fat	Protein	Cals

Mediterranean *Recipe*

RECIPE NAME:

	Mediterranean	Low Carb	Paleo	Vegetarian	Vegan	Dairy Free	Gluten Free
	☐	☐	☐	☐	☐	☐	☐

QTY	INGREDIENTS	RECIPE INSTRUCTIONS

NOTES & RECIPE REVIEW	
	Serves	
	Prep Time	
	Cook Time	
	Tools	
	Temp	

Total	Carbs	Fat	Protein	Cals

Mediterranean *Recipe*

RECIPE NAME:

Mediterranean	Low Carb	Paleo	Vegetarian	Vegan	Dairy Free	Gluten Free
☐	☐	☐	☐	☐	☐	☐

QTY	INGREDIENTS

RECIPE INSTRUCTIONS

NOTES & RECIPE REVIEW

Serves	
Prep Time	
Cook Time	
Tools	
Temp	

Total	Carbs	Fat	Protein	Cals

Mediterranean *Recipe*

RECIPE NAME:

	Mediterranean	Low Carb	Paleo	Vegetarian	Vegan	Dairy Free	Gluten Free
	☐	☐	☐	☐	☐	☐	☐

QTY	INGREDIENTS	RECIPE INSTRUCTIONS

NOTES & RECIPE REVIEW	
	Serves	
	Prep Time	
	Cook Time	
	Tools	
	Temp	

Total	Carbs	Fat	Protein	Cals

Mediterranean *Recipe*

RECIPE NAME:

Mediterranean	Low Carb	Paleo	Vegetarian	Vegan	Dairy Free	Gluten Free
☐	☐	☐	☐	☐	☐	☐

QTY	INGREDIENTS

RECIPE INSTRUCTIONS

NOTES & RECIPE REVIEW

Serves	
Prep Time	
Cook Time	
Tools	
Temp	

Total	Carbs	Fat	Protein	Cals

Mediterranean *Recipe*

RECIPE NAME:

Mediterranean	Low Carb	Paleo	Vegetarian	Vegan	Dairy Free	Gluten Free
☐	☐	☐	☐	☐	☐	☐

QTY	INGREDIENTS	RECIPE INSTRUCTIONS

NOTES & RECIPE REVIEW

Serves	
Prep Time	
Cook Time	
Tools	
Temp	

Total	Carbs	Fat	Protein	Cals

Mediterranean *Recipe*

RECIPE NAME:

	Mediterranean	Low Carb	Paleo	Vegetarian	Vegan	Dairy Free	Gluten Free
	☐	☐	☐	☐	☐	☐	☐

QTY	INGREDIENTS

RECIPE INSTRUCTIONS

NOTES & RECIPE REVIEW

Serves	
Prep Time	
Cook Time	
Tools	
Temp	

	Carbs	Fat	Protein	Cals
Total				

Mediterranean *Recipe*

RECIPE NAME:
_____

	Mediterranean	Low Carb	Paleo	Vegetarian	Vegan	Dairy Free	Gluten Free
	☐	☐	☐	☐	☐	☐	☐

QTY	INGREDIENTS

RECIPE INSTRUCTIONS

NOTES & RECIPE REVIEW

Serves	
Prep Time	
Cook Time	
Tools	
Temp	

Total	Carbs	Fat	Protein	Cals

Mediterranean *Recipe*

RECIPE NAME:

	Mediterranean	Low Carb	Paleo	Vegetarian	Vegan	Dairy Free	Gluten Free
	☐	☐	☐	☐	☐	☐	☐

QTY	INGREDIENTS	RECIPE INSTRUCTIONS

NOTES & RECIPE REVIEW

Serves	
Prep Time	
Cook Time	
Tools	
Temp	

Total	Carbs	Fat	Protein	Cals

Mediterranean Recipe

RECIPE NAME:
_____

Mediterranean	Low Carb	Paleo	Vegetarian	Vegan	Dairy Free	Gluten Free
☐	☐	☐	☐	☐	☐	☐

QTY	INGREDIENTS	RECIPE INSTRUCTIONS

NOTES & RECIPE REVIEW

Serves	
Prep Time	
Cook Time	
Tools	
Temp	

Total	Carbs	Fat	Protein	Cals

Mediterranean *Recipe*

RECIPE NAME:

Mediterranean	Low Carb	Paleo	Vegetarian	Vegan	Dairy Free	Gluten Free
☐	☐	☐	☐	☐	☐	☐

QTY	INGREDIENTS

RECIPE INSTRUCTIONS

NOTES & RECIPE REVIEW

Serves	
Prep Time	
Cook Time	
Tools	
Temp	

Total	Carbs	Fat	Protein	Cals

Mediterranean Recipe

RECIPE NAME:

	Mediterranean	Low Carb	Paleo	Vegetarian	Vegan	Dairy Free	Gluten Free
	☐	☐	☐	☐	☐	☐	☐

QTY	INGREDIENTS	RECIPE INSTRUCTIONS

NOTES & RECIPE REVIEW

Serves	
Prep Time	
Cook Time	
Tools	
Temp	

Total	Carbs	Fat	Protein	Cals

Mediterranean *Recipe*

RECIPE NAME:

	Mediterranean	Low Carb	Paleo	Vegetarian	Vegan	Dairy Free	Gluten Free
	☐	☐	☐	☐	☐	☐	☐

QTY	INGREDIENTS

RECIPE INSTRUCTIONS

NOTES & RECIPE REVIEW

Serves	
Prep Time	
Cook Time	
Tools	
Temp	

Total	Carbs	Fat	Protein	Cals

Mediterranean *Recipe*

RECIPE NAME:

	Mediterranean	Low Carb	Paleo	Vegetarian	Vegan	Dairy Free	Gluten Free
	☐	☐	☐	☐	☐	☐	☐

QTY	INGREDIENTS	RECIPE INSTRUCTIONS

NOTES & RECIPE REVIEW

Serves	
Prep Time	
Cook Time	
Tools	
Temp	

Total	Carbs	Fat	Protein	Cals

Mediterranean *Recipe*

RECIPE NAME:

Mediterranean	Low Carb	Paleo	Vegetarian	Vegan	Dairy Free	Gluten Free
☐	☐	☐	☐	☐	☐	☐

QTY	INGREDIENTS

RECIPE INSTRUCTIONS

NOTES & RECIPE REVIEW

Serves	
Prep Time	
Cook Time	
Tools	
Temp	

Total	Carbs	Fat	Protein	Cals

Mediterranean Recipe

RECIPE NAME:

	Mediterranean	Low Carb	Paleo	Vegetarian	Vegan	Dairy Free	Gluten Free
	☐	☐	☐	☐	☐	☐	☐

QTY	INGREDIENTS	RECIPE INSTRUCTIONS

NOTES & RECIPE REVIEW

Serves	
Prep Time	
Cook Time	
Tools	
Temp	

Total	Carbs	Fat	Protein	Cals

Mediterranean *Recipe*

RECIPE NAME:

	Mediterranean	Low Carb	Paleo	Vegetarian	Vegan	Dairy Free	Gluten Free
	☐	☐	☐	☐	☐	☐	☐

QTY	INGREDIENTS

RECIPE INSTRUCTIONS

NOTES & RECIPE REVIEW

Serves	
Prep Time	
Cook Time	
Tools	
Temp	

Total	Carbs	Fat	Protein	Cals

Mediterranean Recipe

RECIPE NAME:

Mediterranean	Low Carb	Paleo	Vegetarian	Vegan	Dairy Free	Gluten Free
☐	☐	☐	☐	☐	☐	☐

QTY	INGREDIENTS	RECIPE INSTRUCTIONS

NOTES & RECIPE REVIEW

Serves	
Prep Time	
Cook Time	
Tools	
Temp	

Total	Carbs	Fat	Protein	Cals

Mediterranean *Recipe*

RECIPE NAME:

	Mediterranean	Low Carb	Paleo	Vegetarian	Vegan	Dairy Free	Gluten Free
	☐	☐	☐	☐	☐	☐	☐

QTY	INGREDIENTS

RECIPE INSTRUCTIONS

NOTES & RECIPE REVIEW

Serves	
Prep Time	
Cook Time	
Tools	
Temp	

Total	Carbs	Fat	Protein	Cals

Mediterranean *Recipe*

RECIPE NAME:

	Mediterranean	Low Carb	Paleo	Vegetarian	Vegan	Dairy Free	Gluten Free
	☐	☐	☐	☐	☐	☐	☐

QTY	INGREDIENTS

RECIPE INSTRUCTIONS

NOTES & RECIPE REVIEW

Serves	
Prep Time	
Cook Time	
Tools	
Temp	

Total	Carbs	Fat	Protein	Cals

Mediterranean *Recipe*

RECIPE NAME:

	Mediterrane an	Low Carb	Paleo	Vegetarian	Vegan	Dairy Free	Gluten Free
	☐	☐	☐	☐	☐	☐	☐

QTY	INGREDIENTS	RECIPE INSTRUCTIONS

NOTES & RECIPE REVIEW

Serves	
Prep Time	
Cook Time	
Tools	
Temp	

Total	Carbs	Fat	Protein	Cals

Mediterranean *Recipe*

RECIPE NAME:

	Mediterranean	Low Carb	Paleo	Vegetarian	Vegan	Dairy Free	Gluten Free
	☐	☐	☐	☐	☐	☐	☐

QTY	INGREDIENTS	RECIPE INSTRUCTIONS

NOTES & RECIPE REVIEW	
	Serves	
	Prep Time	
	Cook Time	
	Tools	
	Temp	

Total	Carbs	Fat	Protein	Cals

Mediterranean *Recipe*

RECIPE NAME:

	Mediterranean	Low Carb	Paleo	Vegetarian	Vegan	Dairy Free	Gluten Free
	☐	☐	☐	☐	☐	☐	☐

QTY	INGREDIENTS	RECIPE INSTRUCTIONS

NOTES & RECIPE REVIEW

Serves	
Prep Time	
Cook Time	
Tools	
Temp	

Total	Carbs	Fat	Protein	Cals

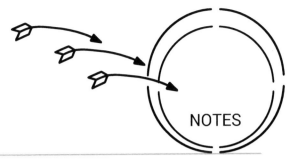

NOTES

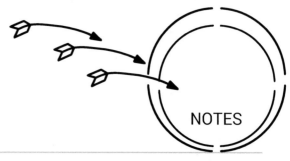

NOTES

Made in United States
Troutdale, OR
12/20/2023